MW01006534

The Effective Preceptor Handbook *for* Nurses

The pocket companion for effective preceptors

DIANA SWIHART PHD, DMIN, MSN, APN CS, RN-BC

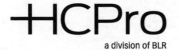

a division of BLR

The Effective Preceptor Handbook for Nurses is published by HCPro, a division of BLR.

Download the additional materials of this book at *www.hcpro.com/downloads/11883.*

ISBN: 978-1-61569-332-0

HCPro provides information resources for the healthcare industry.

HCPro is not affiliated in any way with The Joint Commission, which owns the JCAHO and Joint Commission trademarks.

MAGNET™, MAGNET RECOGNITION PROGRAM®, and ANCC MAGNET RECOGNITION® are trademarks of the American Nurses Credentialing Center (ANCC). The products and services of HCPro are neither sponsored nor endorsed by the ANCC. The acronym "MRP" is not a trademark of HCPro or its parent company.

Diana Swihart, PhD, DMin, MSN, APN CS, RN-BC, Author
Claudette Moore, Acquisitions Editor
Rebecca Hendren, Product Manager
Erin Callahan, Senior Director, Product
Vicki McMahan, Sr. Graphic Designer
Shane Katz, Cover Designer
Jason Gregory, Graphic Design/Layout
Matt Sharpe, Production Supervisor

Advice given is general. Readers should consult professional counsel for specific legal, ethical, or clinical questions.

Arrangements can be made for quantity discounts. For more information, contact:
    HCPro
    75 Sylvan Street, Suite A-101
    Danvers, MA 01923
    Telephone: 800/650-6787 or 781/639-1872
    Fax: 800/639-8511
    E-mail: *customerservice@hcpro.com*

Visit HCPro online at:
www.hcpro.com and *www.hcmarketplace.com*

Dedication

To my beloved husband, Dr. Stan, who is still my greatest encourager and support; to my amazing son Matthew, a brilliant and creative writer in his own genres; and, to my beautiful and gifted daughter-in-law, Gianna, an exceptional nurse serving so many through the American Red Cross. These three are my greatest blessings and the inspiration for all I do. I pray that each and every one of you reading this work have such wondrous blessings in your own lives and careers.

Special Dedication To those who, like my precious Gianna, have the passion and willingness to give back to others; those who understand the importance of giving. Judie Bopp best expressed the specialty of preceptoring and its impact on those who give and receive within the context of such relationships: "The capacity to watch over and guard the well-being of others is an important gift, and one that is learned with great difficulty. For it is one thing to see the situation others are in, but it is quite another to care enough about them to want to help, and yet another to know what to do."

Contents

About the Author

Diana Swihart, PhD, DMin, MSN, APN CS, RN-BC

Dr. Diana Swihart enjoys many roles in her professional career, practicing in widely diverse clinical and nonclinical settings. She is a health care educator and consultant. An author, speaker, researcher, educator, mentor, and consultant, she holds graduate degrees in nursing and leadership and doctorates in theology, ministry, and ancient Near Eastern studies (archaeology). She has provided operational leadership for the preceptorships and shared governance processes for multiple organizations nationally and internationally and facilitated the application of evidence-based practice and nursing research. Dr. Swihart is a member of Sigma Theta Tau International, the National Organization of VA Nurses, the Veterans Educators Integrated Network, and the VHA DoD Facility Based Educators Community of Practice and serves on several professional advisory boards, e.g., Forum for Shared Governance. She also served multiple terms as an American Nurses Credentialing Center (ANCC) Magnet® Appraiser, Treasurer for the National Nursing Staff Development Organization (NNSDO; now the Association for Nursing Professional Development, [ANPD]), as a Member of the Advisory Board of the *Journal of Nursing Regulation*, and as an ANCC Accreditation Commissioner.

Dr. Swihart is the founder and CEO for the American Academy for Preceptor Advancement *(www.preceptoracademy.com)* and has published and spoken on a number of topics related to building effective preceptorships, nursing, shared governance, competency assessment, professional development *(e.g., Nursing Professional Development Review Course* for Gannett Education), and servant leadership, Magnet Recognition Program®, and research- and evidence-based practice at points of service locally, nationally, and internationally. She published *Shared Governance: A Practical Guide for Reshaping Professional Nursing Practice* in 2006 and *Shared Governance: A Practical Approach to Transform Professional Nursing Practice* (2nd ed.) in 2011. In 2008, her publication *Nurse Preceptor Program Builder: Tools for a Successful Preceptor Program* (2nd ed.) was selected as a foundational resource for the national *VHA RN Residency Program*.

Dr. Swihart's training and experiences, including those in academia and staff development, give her a broad and balanced perspective that influences and colors all that she does as she creatively challenges and encourages others to embrace change, shift paradigms, and throw away *the box*.

Acknowledgments

Every work, regardless of scope and size, is completed only with the help and inspiration of others. My utmost appreciation goes to **my beloved family** for their constant support and encouragement, their unwavering belief in me.

I would also like to thank **the preceptors**, those clinicians, educators, and nursing professional development and staff development specialists whose unfailing commitment have provided a legacy of lived experiences in preceptoring and mentoring through transformational leadership to all those they serve.

Finally, I would also like to acknowledge those **speakers and teachers** who have contributed their ideas, lessons learned, and thoughts through the countless classes, seminars, and lectures I have attended over the years. I write from their influence and want to recognize their contributions, though their names are too numerous to list.

—*Dr. Diana Swihart*

Preface

The role of the nurse preceptor, with all of its intrinsic complexities, responsibilities, and accountabilities, is not one to be accepted lightly. Preceptors provide practical and pragmatic support, guiding new employees, new graduates, and students through the onboarding and competency validation processes. As a nurse preceptor, you have the opportunity to help shape their experiences in positive and creative ways. But to do that successfully, you need some tools.

The Effective Preceptor Handbook for Nurses is a compilation of tools to help you develop your professional skills as you advance your understanding of your preceptor roles, competencies, and responsibilities. There are guides for exploring how adults learn, creating a climate of learning, and validating competencies. You can explore ways for providing feedback positively and constructively and evaluating your preceptees and preceptorship. Confronting reality shock and "letting go" of the preceptee as he or she transitions into practice can be difficult for both the preceptor and preceptee. This handbook helps you through both as you grow and develop your knowledge, skills, and abilities in the specialty of preceptoring. These tools can support your work as you participate in a partnership with your leadership, educators, interprofessional colleagues and interdisciplinary team members to ensure your preceptees confidently engage in safe, competent practice.

The information presented in this handbook for nurse preceptors reflects the research and opinions of the author, contributors, and advisors. Because of ongoing research and improvements in preceptoring, information technology, and education, this information, these tools, and their applications are constantly shifting, changing, and evolving as preceptoring continues to grow as a specialty role in healthcare, leadership, and other services and disciplines. It is the author's sincere hope you will add this work to your toolbox and consider how you, too, might contribute to this growing body of knowledge and expertise through your own practice and career development through preceptoring.

Introduction

Few things help an individual more than to
place responsibility upon him, and to
let him know that you trust him.
—*Booker T. Washington*

Being a preceptor has never been easy. Being a nurse preceptor is even more complex and demanding now as the world of nursing becomes increasingly multifaceted and complicated. Practicing nurses assume many more roles and responsibilities, including those of preceptoring. However, you've chosen to be a nurse preceptor. How does that work if the preceptoring duties are separate from other activities, though?

A formal preceptorship is not just another situation where your duties and responsibilities are multiplied. As a nurse preceptor, you are generally most effective when working in a structured program with time allocated apart from other duties to preceptor new employees or students and validate preceptee competencies.

Effective, committed preceptors play a major role in improving the retention of new nurses and encouraging students in the profession of nursing. Nurse preceptors such as you are nurses who can talk about difficulties they have met, share insights they have gained, and pass on lessons they have learned by caring for patients in the many arenas of need they encounter each day. The right preceptor can help the new nurse or graduate to overcome the hurdles of new technology, inadequate staffing, complicated medical interventions, and complex diagnoses.

Preceptors facilitate the orientation, growth, and development of nurses who will one day work side by side with them and who will eventually become their peers, colleagues, and leaders. Staff nurses who assume the roles and responsibilities of a preceptor can connect with new hires, students, new graduate nurses (preceptees), and the newly qualified in ways that no one else can, building trust and responsibility as they gently draw their preceptees into the "real world" of healthcare.

Who really benefits from all of this effort? Patients—and us! Effective nurse preceptorships create an environment to build the close, trusting relationships needed to develop preceptees to their fullest potential.

Use this handbook as a road map. It will provide you with the background necessary to help the new hire, student, new graduate nurse, and the newly qualified examine and apply nursing theory and evidence-based practice (EBP) in clinical settings. You will increase your preceptees' personal and professional growth and ease their transition into professional practice. Additional tools available from HCPro that can help you create your program include *The Preceptor Program Builder,* and *The Preceptee Handbook,* available on *www.hcmarketplace.com.*

As you begin, establish the relationship, review the objectives and the duration and termination of the program, and address the expectations of the preceptorship. This is an excellent time to consider creating a professional portfolio if the preceptee does not already have one. If he or she does have a portfolio, review it together and discuss how to add to it during the onboarding and competency validation processes.

Preceptor Roles, Competencies, and Responsibilities

If I am walking with two other men,
each of them will serve
as my teacher.
I will pick out the good points of the
one and imitate them, and
the bad points of
the other and correct them in myself.
—Confucius, Chinese philosopher, teacher (551–479 BC)

The first step to becoming a professional nurse preceptor is to understand the essential roles, responsibilities, and accountabilities of the preceptor and preceptee within the context of their relationship.

Preceptors are experienced and competent staff nurses who have received formal training to function in this capacity and who serve as role models and resource people to preceptees. They merge the knowledge, skills, abilities, and roles of both coaches and mentors to help preceptees develop and mature into strong practicing professionals within new professional practice environments.

A preceptor is a

Servant leader	Recordkeeper
Educator/teacher	Evaluator
Coach	Advocate
Encourager	Role model
Socializer	Mentor

Preceptors are staff nurses who generally have more work experience and knowledge of the organization and unit, are dedicated to helping other nurses advance in their careers, provide feedback on preceptees' strengths and weaknesses, and offer suggestions for improvement in tasks and behaviors. Preceptors help preceptees balance tasks with work issues (e.g., time management, accepting new responsibilities, adjusting to a new work environment and team, stress management, and how to give and receive constructive criticism).

Other roles you will play as an effective preceptor include the following:

- Providing leadership, guidance, and support
- Modeling desired skills and behaviors
- Listening and communicating with empathy and patience
- Providing organization and unit information
- Managing the preceptee's orientation and competencies

Preceptor competencies

How do you develop your competencies as a preceptor? By practicing the specialty of preceptoring. Preceptor competencies emerge from identified standards of practice, conceptualized in diverse roles and multidimensional functions. Each dimension supports the development and maintenance of competencies at all points of service beginning with where you are in your knowledge, skills, and practice and taking them as far as you choose to go. Competencies develop, grow, and change over time as you engage in activities that prepare you to fulfill the specialty role of "preceptor."

Some ways to identify and develop your preceptor competencies include the following:

- Maintain professional knowledge and skills necessary to help preceptees acclimate to specific areas of professional practice
- Relate established expectations to your own levels of performance
- Engage in self-assessment to identify strengths and opportunities for growth
- Participate in learning activities to meet identified opportunities for growth and support for functioning in your preceptor role
- Identify organizational support available when fulfilling your preceptor role
- Exhibit effective communication skills and a state of open-mindedness
- Establish collegial relationships with members of the workforce team

Essential expectations and responsibilities

If you are to become a truly effective preceptor, you must be willing to take on the following 12 essential responsibilities:

1. **Orient your preceptee to the nursing unit.** Begin by introducing yourself to your preceptees and reviewing the orientation,

competency assessment, and competency verification process-es with them. Talk about yourselves and get to know each other. If you have attended a preceptor program that used the Preceptor Workbook, complete the preceptor and preceptee questionnaire together to help you get to know one another. This will help you be more sensitive to the unique concerns and needs of your preceptees and be more successful in meet-ing the goals of the preceptorships. Examples of ways to begin this initial orientation to the new nursing unit to help your preceptee engage quickly include the following:

- Introduce the preceptee to other staff members
- Show the preceptee around, where to put his or her things, and so on
- Describe the chain of command
- Talk about what's happening in the assigned work area
- Be positive—stay with the preceptee
- Put yourself in his or her position; remember what it was like to be "new"
- Practice whatever you preach
- Initiate the orientation and competency assessment processes

2. **Facilitate the learning experience.** Begin by reflecting on your own behaviors, skills, abilities, and attitudes. Consider what you want to accomplish through the preceptorship, and if you attended a preceptor program that used the Preceptor Workbook, complete the preceptor development plan.

Facilitating learning is not the same as learning and applied learning, e.g., being told how to give an injection is not the same thing as understanding the process and rationale for it, actually doing an injection on a patient, and documenting the medication administration in a patient record. Facilitating learning in preceptorships means that you provide the support and practice opportunities that will help your preceptee come to work with a positive attitude, to safely and accurately practice their skills until they are mastered, and to develop and model professional behaviors.

Your preceptees need your support and encouragement to apply the things you are teaching them during orientation as well as when verifying competencies. They draw on many academic and life experiences to form their beliefs and expectations about what constitutes excellence in nursing. You provide the support, advocacy, parameters, and setting for them to achieve what they have learned. As evidence of those achievements, you will help them create a portfolio to showcase their successes.

3. **Establish the schedule for your preceptee.** Prepare your schedule for the anticipated length of the preceptorship with your preceptee and any input from the manager or supervisor. Be sure to address some of the following considerations:

   • Discuss any potential scheduling conflicts and ensure you will spend as much time with the preceptee as possible.

   • Identify a backup preceptor (assistant or secondary preceptor, preferably one with training/experience as a preceptor) for those shifts, tours of duty, or limited times when your schedule conflicts with that of your preceptee.

- Do *not* allow preceptees to be added to the assigned staffing mix until the preceptorship and clinical or service orientation have been completed. It is your role as preceptor to protect and advocate for the preceptee in such situations whenever necessary.

4. **Guide your preceptee during clinical practice.** You may need to provide direct guidance during the orientation and when verifying competencies for the preceptees to:
   - Demonstrate nursing skills and techniques
   - Supervise clinical practice
   - Intervene only in an emergent situation in which there may be a danger to a patient
   - Assess and verify competencies

Continuously assess where your preceptees are in the preceptorship. Revise the orientation to reflect their changing needs. Some new nurses are seasoned practitioners and may require only minimal guidance. Student nurses and new nurse graduates often bring life experiences and past professional roles to their clinical positions. Still other preceptees may have difficulty changing methods of practice to reflect their new expectations. Give them respectful guidance:

- Do not assume that preceptees are familiar with the clinical setting or the situation. Discuss what they know before deciding what they need.
- Ask questions to confirm comprehension and perceptions— yours and theirs—and to generate further discussion. Case studies, debriefings, reflective practice, and shared stories are excellent tools for giving directions and encouragement, verifying competency, and redirecting behaviors.

- Include explanations as you go. Preceptees respond more positively and effectively when they understand from the onset why they are doing the requested tasks, abilities, or behaviors.

5. **Supervise competency assessment and verification during preceptorship.** Competency assessment and verification are generally specific to the needs of the preceptee. Make sure you allow your preceptees to assist in deciding what work-based competencies need to be addressed besides those required for new hires to meet organizational and service-specific goals. Engage your preceptee in reflective discussion to:

- Select competencies that matter to the new employee or student, your preceptee. Choose assignments that will give him or her opportunities to demonstrate those competencies.

- Select the correct verification method (tests/exams, return demonstrations, evidences of daily work, case studies, exemplars, peer reviews, self-assessments, discussion/ reflection groups, presentations, mock events/surveys, quality improvement monitors) for each identified competency.

- Clarify the responsibility and accountability of the preceptor, preceptee, educator, and manager or supervisor in the competency process.

- Implement a preceptee-centered verification process in which the preceptee has choices from among a number of verification methods for the identified competencies.

- Differentiate what is a competency deficit versus what is a compliance issue.

- Promptly and efficiently address any deficits and performance problems with the preceptee as soon as they are identified.

6. **Teach new skills and reinforce previous learning.** Establish what your preceptees already know or can do; demonstrate the new skills, knowledge, or abilities; have preceptees perform any return demonstrations, if necessary; and evaluate the outcomes when the new knowledge, skill, or ability is applied in practice during the preceptorship.

7. **Gradually increase your preceptee's responsibility for patient care.** Preceptees often require three to six months, and sometimes as much as one year, to be fully integrated into the culture of the new organization. Orientations usually range from a few days to four to six weeks, depending on the organization and the resources available for new employees. The following considerations are an important part of your planning process:
   - Discuss the amount of time available for the preceptorship with preceptees and nurse managers.
   - Assess preceptees' clinical orientation and competency verification needs and assign increasing responsibilities as they become more proficient and confident in their abilities to practice safely and effectively in their new positions.
   - Help preceptees set priorities, establish daily goals, manage time, delegate appropriately, and communicate professionally with other team members as you gradually introduce new and more challenging patient care assignments.

8. **Provide timely feedback to your preceptee regarding all aspects of clinical practice.** You must give consistent, fair,

honest, and timely verbal and written feedback to your preceptees often. This feedback serves three primary purposes:

- To reinforce positive behavior
- To promptly address inappropriate behaviors
- To build confidence and self-efficacy

9. **Serve as a role model for your preceptee during clinical
   experiences.** This may be your greatest challenge as a preceptor. Subtle techniques that can help you serve as a consistent
   role model for your preceptees include the following:

- Dress professionally. Maintain clean and appropriate
  uniforms, if applicable.
- Be prompt and timely, and maintain excellent attendance.
  Arrive before your preceptee.
- Be prepared for report and participate if applicable.
- Follow nursing service policies and procedures at all times.
- Be courteous and respectful of all team members and
  leadership at all times, especially when you disagree with
  their decisions or abilities.
- Stay positive and enthusiastic about professional nursing
  but realistic in recognizing limitations and areas for
  improvement.
- Maintain your membership and activities in professional
  organizations and affiliations.

10. **Work closely with nursing faculty, staff development spe-
    cialists, and/or hospital educators to identify education
    gaps and learning opportunities.** Use your available human
    resources—internal and external stakeholders, clinical educa-
    tors, advanced practice nurses, pharmacists, biomedical staff,

informatics staff, housekeepers, students, college or university partners, community members—to provide more complex and integrated training opportunities. As the preceptor, you will coordinate the preceptees' learning activities with the appropriate resources and verify the preceptees' competencies with patient care outcomes.

11. **Plan specific learning experiences that correlate with unit competencies and clinical objectives.** Ensure that your preceptees have as many opportunities for supervised practice for the wide variety of skills, knowledge, and abilities as they need to be successful in the assigned position and nursing unit. Be particularly careful to verify competencies in any skill with potential patient outcomes that are high risk (have a high probability of causing potential harm to the patient or preceptee) and time-sensitive (there would be no time to call for help or look up the procedure first). Mock events and return demonstrations are helpful in providing practice and in verifying such competencies.

12. **Complete all necessary paperwork related to the preceptorship.** Complete preceptor/preceptee questionnaires and forms, skills checklists, orientation forms, competency verification forms, feedback, and evaluations in a timely manner. Review all appropriate documents with the preceptee, the clinical nurse educator and hospital educator, and the nurse manager. Maintain careful records in a secure area. Remember, these always have some information that neither you nor your preceptees may want to share with others.

How Adults Learn

Education is the kindling of the flame,
not the filling of the vessel.
—*Socrates*

Preceptees come to the preceptoring relationship as adult learners
seeking to increase their knowledge, skills, and abilities (cognitive,
psychomotor, and affective learning domains) in new and changing
professional practice settings. The preceptee's goal is to successfully
complete his or her orientation and competency verification
periods. As a preceptor, you are a role model who possesses the
knowledge and experience necessary to help the preceptee meet
that goal.

Effective facilitation occurs when preceptors understand adult
learning principles and encourage preceptees to be creative and
independent in meeting their orientation and competency require-
ments, to think critically, and to formulate their own professional
strengths and abilities. Preceptors establish rapport with preceptees
by acknowledging their lived experiences, thoughts, and feelings
about matters related to patient assignments, activities, policies,
and other concerns and encouraging them to ask questions and to
express personal viewpoints.

As a preceptor facilitating the learning process with your preceptees, you will need to consider several major questions:

- What is to be learned from the preceptee's assignment or
  experience?
- What knowledge, skills, or abilities are "need to know" versus
  "nice to know?"
- How is the information to be used or implemented?
- How and when is the learning to be accomplished?
- How is the learning to be communicated and documented?
- How is the learning to be evaluated?
- How can the preceptor facilitate the learning?

How adults access and process information

When communication breaks down between preceptors and
preceptees, the problem may not be resistance or incompetence, for
example. Preceptors may assume that preceptees will receive and
interpret information in the same way they do. When this does not
happen, preceptors may assume there is something wrong with the
preceptee. This faulty perception creates conflict in their communication and relationship when the problem may simply be a matter
of differences in how each one accesses and processes information
(Meier 2000; Russell 1999). Preceptors will add significantly to the
success of the preceptoring relationship by understanding something about teaching and learning effectiveness as they relate to
these differences and learning how to navigate them accurately.

Accessing information through learning styles

To understand how to teach others, you must understand the variety
of ways in which people learn. *The learning style inventory* in Figure
1 will provide some insight into how you and your preceptees prefer

to access information. The best learning and applications to practice occur when all learning styles are used together.

There are four primary ways that adults prefer to access information: visual, auditory, kinesthetic, and intellectual (reflective). The learning style inventory provides some insight into how you and your preceptees prefer to access information. The best learning and application to practice occurs when all four learning styles are used together. Are you a visual, auditory, or kinesthetic (tactile) learner? Do you see the implications that each learning style may have for how preceptees access information during the orientation and competency verification process?

Figure 1: Learning style inventory

Learning style	Implications and strategies for preceptors
Visual Learning by seeing, observing, and picturing things and events. There is more equipment in humans for processing visual information than for any other sense. Most people are visual learners. Research demonstrates that mental imagery increases learning ~12% on immediate recall and ~26% on long-term retention regardless of age, ethnicity, gender, or preferred learning style (Meier 2000). Preceptees think and communicate in pictures and multiple dimensions.	Preceptees learn best when they can see real-world examples, diagrams, idea maps, icons, pictures, and images of all kinds while they are learning. They use peripheral learning objects (e.g., bulletin boards, wall maps and diagrams, and unit dashboards). They ask learners to observe a clinical situation, and then to think and talk about it, drawing out the processes, principles, or meanings it illustrated. Appeal to these preceptees by: - adding visual words to describe what things look like - drawing pictures to illustrate your points - bringing color teaching and orientation materials - writing things down for them - providing charts and diagrams - practicing doodling while they speak; learning to draw

Figure 1: Learning style inventory, cont'd

Learning style	Implications and strategies for preceptors
Auditory Learning by talking, hearing, and reading, especially out loud. All learners, particularly strong auditory ones, learn by sounds, dialog, reading out loud, telling someone out loud what they just experienced, heard, or learned, talking to themselves, remembering jingles and rhymes, listening to audio cassettes, and repeating sounds in their heads.	Have preceptees read out loud, one paragraph at a time, and paraphrasing it. Have them tell stories with embedded information (e.g., case studies, reflective discussion). Pair preceptees with staff members. Let preceptees describe what they learned and how they might apply it. Have them practice a skill and describe in detail what is being done. Ask preceptees to talk nonstop while problem-solving. Appeal to these preceptees by: - making eye contact - slowing down your speech - keeping control of your body language - resisting the urge to draw or write - pausing - resisting the urge to interrupt
Kinesthetic (or somatic) Learning by actively moving and doing, engaging the body (somatic) in the learning process. These learners often cannot sit still, must move their bodies to keep their minds alive and active, and prefer hands-on learning activities. Sometimes these preceptees may be considered disruptive or hyperactive, inattentive and disrespectful of the preceptor's attempts to explain details or review lengthy policies and procedures. It is important for the preceptor to understand that for preceptees who prefer to access information kinesthetically, inhibiting them from using their bodies in learning also interferes with their ability to fully engage their minds.	Don't just sit there, *do* something! Get the body involved in activities. Have preceptees practice techniques, perform procedures, do an active learning exercise, or complete a project that requires physical activity. If part of the orientation is classroom-based, allow these preceptees frequent breaks and permission to get up during classes and walk about in the back of the room. Limit distractions to preceptees who might be present and have different learning styles by managing the types of activities and learning environments chosen for the orientation and competency verifications. Appeal to these preceptees by: - allowing them to multitask - asking them to talk - interrupting them to move faster - giving them something to take with them - keeping the lights on for a presentation (during orientation, for example) - asking about and talking about emotions

Figure 1: Learning style inventory, cont'd

Learning style	Implications and strategies for preceptors
Intellectual Learning by critical thinking, problem-solving, and reflecting—what learners do in their minds internally as they exercise their intelligence to reflect on experience and to create connections, meanings, plans, and values out of it; the reflecting, creating, problem-solving part of a person. This process connects the body's mental, physical, emotional, and intuitive experiences to build fresh meaning. To some degree, all preceptors and preceptees engage this learning style. It is the sense-maker of the mind, how people "think," integrate experience, create new neural networks, and learn. This is how preceptees turn experience into knowledge, knowledge into understanding, and understanding into wisdom.	These preceptees may need to receive the information and have time to reflect on it, to mentally pull it apart and restructure it before they can accept this learning for application. Give preceptees orientations and competency verification methods that involve the following: - Solving problems - Formulating questions - Analyzing experiences - Applying new ideas to work - Doing strategic planning - Creating personal meaning - Generating creative ideas - Thinking through implications of ideas - Accessing and distilling information - Creating mental models

Processing information through multiple intelligences

Multiple intelligences (MI) are mapped to competencies preceptees use to process information (Russell 1999; Gardner 1993). Preceptees may prefer certain MIs, usually those valued by their culture and family. These MIs are strengths that preceptees default to when they are being creative or solving problems.

Ten categories, or aptitudes, MIs, are mapped to competencies people use to process information:

1. Interpersonal intelligence

2. Logical and mathematical intelligence

3. Spatial and visual intelligence

4. Musical intelligence

5. Linguistic and verbal intelligence

6. Intrapersonal intelligence

7. Bodily and kinesthetic intelligence

8. Emotional intelligence

9. Naturalist intelligence

10. Existential and spiritual intelligence

MIs correspond to learning styles in how people prefer to manage information. Keep in mind the following overlaps when preparing your teaching and learning strategies for preceptees:

Multiple Intelligences	Learning Styles
Bodily/kinesthetic, emotional	kinesthetic/tactile
Linguistic/verbal, musical, existential/spiritual	auditory
Spatial/visual, naturalist	visual
Intrapersonal, interpersonal, logical/mathematical, existential/spiritual	intelligent

Every person has access to all 10 MIs for processing information. Choosing to use less-preferred aptitudes will help preceptees develop them and expand their abilities to engage in all aspects of nursing care in the cognitive, psychomotor, and affective domains.

Preceptoring and teaching effectiveness

A basic understanding of policies used within the organization is required of nursing students and new employees. A **visual** learner may be able to read the policies and understand them. An **auditory** learner may need to have the policies read out loud and discussed. A **tactile** learner may have to actually implement the policies— in other words, do something—to fully grasp the policies.

An intelligent learner may need time to reflect on the policies before deciding on how to implement them. These preferences for accessing information (learning styles) are linked to the preceptee's preferences for processing information (MIs).

In the role of preceptor, you will want to select teaching strategies that engage all the preceptee's preferences for accessing and processing information to maximize retention of learning.

Teaching strategies in the three learning domains

There are three learning domains: the cognitive domain, the psychomotor domain, and the affective domain. Each time you begin a teaching session, you must consider the domain or combination of domains in which you are teaching.

Cognitive domain

The **cognitive domain** focuses on preceptees' knowledge and intellectual skills. Teaching strategies include lectures, presentations, tests, case studies, and written materials. Test retention with objective and subjective test items (e.g., ask the preceptee to calculate a drug dose [objective] and choose an accurate pain description on a patient pain scale [subjective]). The cognitive domain addresses the following three instructional levels:

1. **Fact:** Preceptees are asked to recall information; learning objectives use verbs such as define, match, and list

2. **Understanding:** Preceptees join two or more concepts; learning objectives use verbs such as describe, explain, and contrast

3. **Application:** Preceptees merge two or more concepts and apply this knowledge to a new situation; learning objectives use verbs such as apply, demonstrate, and illustrate

Psychomotor domain

The **psychomotor domain** focuses on preceptees' skills and physical abilities. Teaching strategies include performance skill testing, mock events, quality improvement monitors, return demonstrations, and evidence of daily work. The psychomotor domain addresses the following three instructional levels:

1. **Imitation:** Preceptees complete a return demonstration of skill, either under direct supervision of the preceptor or with evidence of daily work (e.g., passing a medication and accurately charting it as evidenced by the chart review and patient's report); learning objectives use verbs such as *follow directions, initiate,* and *carry out*

2. **Practice:** Preceptees have the opportunity to repeat the sequence of events in any procedure as often as needed to build proficiency without direct supervision; learning objectives use verbs and phrases such as *repeat, perform,* and *go through the motion*

3. **Habit:** Preceptees perform the identified skill in twice the time it takes the preceptor to perform it; learning objectives use verbs and phrases such as perform *rapidly, fit action to a new situation,* and *complete smoothly and efficiently*

Affective domain

The **affective domain** focuses on preceptees' emotionally based behaviors. Teaching strategies include reflective exemplars, self-assessments, discussions, storytelling, and peer reviews.

Learning objectives use verbs such as *accept, challenge, defend, dispute, judge, praise, question, support,* and *share.* The affective domain addresses three instructional levels: awareness, distinction, and integration.

Tip

Preceptees bring a uniqueness and variety of characteristics, lived experiences, education, and learning preferences to the practice setting. Preceptors must be innovative, intuitive, and adept at understanding how others manage information to be able to teach preceptees from all three domains (cognitive, psycho-motor, and affective) to successfully transition into their new roles and responsibilities. These are key to helping preceptees understand and apply the content given.

Creating a Climate for Learning

If you are planning for a year, sow rice;
if you are planning for a decade, plant trees;
if you are planning for a lifetime, educate people.
— *Chinese proverb*

Establish a learning climate on the nursing unit, in the service, and across the organization that will help you implement the adult learning principles throughout the orientation and validation processes.

Physical challenges

The unit environment has to be consciously shaped to maximize personal interaction and learning. There must be suitable places for quiet reading, one-on-one discussions, small class settings, and practice space for demonstrations and simulations using mannequins or models. Simulation laboratories, clinical-based competency assessments, primary care settings, critical care practice environments, and other workplaces with complex traffic flow (patients, staff, visitors) and potential for rapid changes (e.g., emergency departments), for example, can be especially challenging for orientation and competency validation.

Preceptoring at points of service also require special consideration when patient acuity levels increase, staffing is limited (e.g., due to sick leave, holidays, reduced staff), and preceptees are needed for patient care instead of orientation or competency validation. At times, preceptors are called on to work shifts or tours of duty that do not coincide with those of their preceptees. These challenges and workplace decisions leave preceptees working alone before they are ready to practice in their new environments of care. In such situations, you must find creative ways to continue your preceptoring activities.

Carefully consider the work environment and the potential for conflicting schedules when developing your preceptorship.

Emotional challenges

The creation of a nonthreatening emotional climate is a little more challenging and can take more time for you to achieve. The emotional climate of the preceptorship should be a comfort zone where everyone understands that every person's views are valued and respected as equal. How each member of the unit staff speaks to others in the group is important, as is full unit participation, for integrating the preceptee into his or her new team.

One way to test the emotional climate is to encourage your preceptee to bring up subjects or ideas for discussion during staff meetings. Can the preceptee share his or her ideas with confidence and security? Empathy and motivation are embedded in how people express their *emotional intelligence*, the ability to identify, understand, and manage emotions in positive ways. How does your preceptee relieve stress, communicate in difficult situations, or handle conflict? Is he or she able to empathize with unlovely or abrasive patients when caring for them? How does he or she interact with others?

Some of the emotional challenges you and your preceptee may encounter may be connected to the level of confidence you have in yourself as a preceptor, in your preceptee as he or she advances through orientation and competency validation, and in the staff as they interact with you and your preceptee. For example, does the staff support the time you spend with your preceptee or do they begrudge you both your partnership and time together? Is your preceptee nervous about his or her new responsibilities? Are you still excited about being a preceptor? When it is time to let go, have you prepared your preceptee to transition into independent practice?

Emotional challenges can be positive and encouraging, as well as troubling or stressful. Explore the emotional needs of both yourself and your preceptee to facilitate self-awareness, insight, empathy, and stress. Develop your ability to manage the challenges emotions can cause in a preceptorship for you as a preceptor, for your preceptee, and for the staff.

Tip

Taking physical and emotional challenges into consideration and addressing them in your teaching and validation processes will develop your skills as preceptor and increase the potential for your preceptees' success.

A nonthreatening and encouraging way to approach such challenges is by helping your preceptee build a professional portfolio. What are some of the physical work environments the preceptee has oriented to before? How has the preceptee managed the stress of school and work prior to coming to this organization, this position? A portfolio offers many opportunities for reflective discussions, to explore the preceptee's current and previous accomplishments, and to plan career goals for future positions and advancement. It acts as a foundation for encouragement and building confidence as the preceptee grows in his or her position and profession. But what if either you or the preceptee has never created a professional portfolio? What would you put into one? Where do you start? Let's begin with your own portfolio.

Building professional portfolios

Portfolios are generally collections of artifacts and documents organized to present the preceptors' knowledge, skills, and achievements. It can be one of the most important tools in your preceptor program. It captures evidence, which is essential to proving value, showing work product, and making it easier for preceptors to repeat what works and adapt what does not work in preceptorships. A *preceptor portfolio* is a collection of all the materials you select or develop as you grow in your specialty roles and accountabilities as a preceptor. It includes information and examples of your education, experiences, and teaching and preceptoring activities relevant to demonstrating your mastery of preceptoring.

Each preceptor's portfolio is unique to him or her. What goes into the portfolio is usually a personal choice. However, some organizations or services may have a template for what they want to see included if the portfolio is used as part of their performance plan or professional development. The portfolio is then updated regularly to reflect the preceptor's growing expertise and to record new activities and achievements.

Portfolios exhibit examples and evidence of your work, skills, and accomplishments that are practical, reflective, and designed to encourage further preceptor development. When determining what to include in your portfolio, consider the list of materials most often found in a preceptor portfolio (see Figure 2) and use the following questions to help guide your decisions.

- Why create a portfolio?

    - To display activities and accomplishments already completed

    - To illustrate the need for additional training and preceptor development

    - To encourage collaboration and discussion to facilitate future activities

- How will you organize your portfolio, e.g., in an electronic folder, binder, or set of regular files?

- How and when will you update your portfolio?

- How will you represent changes as your specialty in preceptoring advances and matures?

Evidence of competency and proficiency need not be limited solely to preceptoring done in a program, during orientation, or in transitioning an employee or student to a new role, for example. The materials included in a portfolio are evidence of competence and proficiency in the specialization of preceptoring, not a listing of how or where you developed them. Simple completion of a course or recitation of information alone is not strong enough evidence.

Portfolio development and evidences of mastery of core competencies in preceptoring provide a more complete assessment of achievement for advancing preceptoring to the level of a specialty. Ask yourself the following questions when creating your preceptor portfolio:

- Do the items in my portfolio work together to provide a comprehensive and coherent picture of my preceptoring abilities and activities?
- Do the items I selected demonstrate my personal and professional development as a preceptor, e.g., certificates and/or certifications in preceptoring?

Figure 2. Materials often included in the preceptor portfolio

Preceptor Portfolio Materials	
• Career summary and goals • Professional philosophy or mission statement • Traditional resume or CV • Scannable, text-based resume or CV • Skills, abilities, and marketable qualities • Samples of your work • Research, publications, reports • Testimonials and letters of recommendations • List of accomplishments • Awards and honors	• Conference and workshops • Transcripts, degrees, licenses, certificates, and certifications (especially certificates and certifications in preceptoring) • Professional development activities • Military records, awards, and badges • Volunteer and community service • References list (those who provide references or letters or recommendations for you)

Source: www.quintcareers.com/ job_search_portfolio.html

Preceptor certificates and certifications

Preceptoring has historically been loosely managed and often just another "duty as assigned." In recent years, though, we have found a growing need for trained preceptors with obligated work time for moving preceptees through orientation and competency validation processes. The knowledge, skills, and abilities of preceptors continue to advance through training, continuing education, and workforce development. Implementing a systematic approach to preceptoring—learning by doing through an apprentice-like process—opens the door for recognition.

Tip

Certification is the process by which a nongovernmental agency or an association grants recognition to an individual who has met certain predetermined qualifications. Certification can be used for employment, validation of competence, recognition of excellence, or regulation of preceptorships. Certification can be mandatory or voluntary. Certification validates an individual's knowledge, skills, and attitudes in a defined role, area of practice, and level of advancement based on predetermined standards.

Certificates for training, education, and program completion have been a standard practice in the preceptoring specialty. Preceptor specialty certification based on a scope and standards of practice for preceptor advancement, like certificates and licenses, are important additions to your portfolio.

Validating Competency

*The most important practical lesson that can be given to
nurses is to teach them what to observe, how to observe, what
symptoms indicate improvement, what the reverse, which
are of importance, which are of none, and which are
evidence of neglect and of what kind of neglect.*
—*Florence Nightingale*

Competency validation is the ultimate goal of the preceptoring
process. Competency-based orientations initiate competency
assessment and verification processes for preceptees during the
orientation.

Competencies can be measured against well-developed professional
standards published by respected organizations (e.g., state boards
of nursing, professional nursing organizations, or The Joint
Commission). They can be improved through training and development. Therefore, one of your major roles as preceptor is to assess
and verify competencies during orientation.

Orientation and verifying competency processes

Competency-based orientations offer numerous advantages for
preceptorships. They give clear guidelines regarding competency

expectations and can decrease the amount of time spent in orientation for more experienced and skilled preceptees, such as those who have worked in the organization and nursing department but recently transferred from another department or unit. Preceptees who have difficulty completing their competencies are quickly identified.

Preceptors can review the competency assessment and verification form used by their organization with preceptees to provide timely feedback on progress and remediate or restructure their clinical experiences to address those deficits or problem areas. Figure 3 provides you with a sample preceptor position description.

The three important elements of competency-based orientations are as follow:

1. **Technical competence.** This is the most familiar and objective skill domain. Elements are traditionally found on checklists, and competency is measured by direct observation of psychomotor tasks. Efficiency components are often added to assess advanced competency. Examples of behaviors used to describe technical competence might include:

   - Start an IV and manage the equipment properly

   - Draw blood from an arterial line

   - Verify accuracy of data transfer

   - Identify problematic lab values and take appropriate actions

   - Respond to STAT orders within 30 minutes

2. **Interpersonal competence.** This skill domain refers to the effective use of interpersonal communication when working

Figure 3: Sample preceptor position description

Position-specific competencies including technical skills

Date of initial assessment _____   Name: _____   Service/Section: _____   Position: _____

Verification: ME/S – Mock event/Survey; **T** – Test/Exam; **SCL** – Skills checklist; **Sim** – Simulation; **Pres** – Presentations/Rounds; **EF** – Employee feedback/Self-assessment; **PR** – Peer review; **RD** – Return demonstration; **P&P** – Policy & procedure review; **EDW** – Evidence of daily work; **CS** – Case studies; **EX** – Exemplars; **QI** – QI monitors; **D/RG** – Discussion/Reflection group

Competency level: E – Education/Training needed; **S** – Competent - Self-directed education/training may be desired; **C** – Competent through education/training/experience verification

COMPETENCY	DESCRIPTION of COMPETENCY (BEHAVIORS)	Competency Level			Demonstrated Competency		Competency verifier's initials	COMMENTS/ EMPLOYEE FEEDBACK (Please state any additional training/experiences you would like and/or need to have)
		E	S	C	Verification methods	Date met		

Overall competency level (circle one):   E   S   C

E – Education/Training needed
S – Competent - Self-directed education/ training may be desired
C – Competent through education/ training/experience

Employee Signature: _____   Date: _____   Verifiers' Signatures: _____   Date: _____
Preceptors' Signatures: _____   Date: _____   Manager/Supervisor Signature: _____   Date: _____

with others. These competencies, too, are often found on checklists and are measured by direct observation of interactions and behaviors that consistently convey caring and courteous attitudes.

- Greet staff, patients, and families with warmth and genuineness.

- Call the patient by his or her preferred name.

- Display proper phone etiquette.

- Anticipate patient and family anxiety; offer information, reassurance, and comfort.

- Work cooperatively with team members.

3. **Critical thinking (or decision-making) competence.** This skill domain addresses preceptees' abilities to apply principles of critical thinking, problem solving, and decision-making to evidence-based practice. To measure competencies in this skill domain, preceptors must be more creative in their verification methods. Competencies are predicated on preceptees' abilities to recognize problems, identify alternative actions, anticipate outcomes, and make choices based on the most current best practices. Asking questions helps them get beneath the surface of problems, generate more questions, and increase the number of possible solutions. Examples of critical-thinking competencies include the ability to:

- Ask "why" questions

- Look for patterns and trends; be open to possibilities

- View events as part of a larger whole

- Use intuition and "hunches" when problem solving

- Seek advice

Questions to Promote Critical Thinking

Preceptorships provide a safe environment during orientation for preceptees to explore the challenging problems found in complex healthcare systems. Guided questions can stimulate critical thinking and enhance preceptees' decision-making skills.

- Given these lab results, how will you change your nursing care plan?
- How will you prioritize your care today?
- What alternative nursing measures would work in this situation?
- What else could be causing your patient's symptoms?
- How will you determine the effectiveness of that intervention?
- How will you document your patient's outcomes related to that treatment?

Do not confuse personality traits or characteristics with competency. They are not performance indicators. The following is a list of some common traits that you should *not* use to evaluate competency:

- Cooperative
- Conforms to policies
- Codependent
- Assertive
- Is a team player
- Flexible
- Aggressive
- Shows initiative
- Passive
- Committed
- Decisive
- Creative

Preceptors frequently need to check their perceptions with their preceptees before making a final decision regarding competency levels of knowledge, skills, and abilities in any skill domain, to ensure objectivity rather than subjectivity. This is critical for accurate feedback and evaluations of the preceptorship and the direct (e.g., preceptor, preceptee) and indirect (e.g., manager or supervisor, educator, staff) participants.

Orientation and competency validation processes are bound up in the policies and protocols of the organization. As a practicing preceptor, build your tasks and activities within the preceptorship around these documents and incorporate the forms and resources of the facility and the nursing service. This will increase your ability to successfully transition your preceptee into the protocols and processes of the organization through onboarding, competency assessment, and consistent feedback.

Providing Feedback

*The single biggest problem in communication
is the illusion that it has taken place.*
—*George Bernard Shaw*

Your preceptee needs daily, accurate feedback on the things he or she is doing well, areas in which additional work is needed, and progress toward goals and objectives.

Feedback must be specific, factual, descriptive, clearly understood by the preceptor and preceptee, timed to be most useful, sensitive to the preceptor and preceptee, constructive, and directed at behavior rather than personality traits. Whenever possible, provide positive feedback. When necessary, provide constructive feedback. Avoid giving negative feedback if at all possible.

Complete the evaluation form you use in your facility at each agreed-upon time interval (e.g., every week during the preceptorship) and at the termination of the preceptoring relationship.

When giving feedback, do the following:

- Describe specifically what was observed—who, what, when, where, and how

- Avoid generalizing or making assumptions
- Relate how the observed behavior or actions made you feel
- Suggest an alternative behavior or action

Continuous feedback allows preceptors to:

- Motivate and positively reinforce learning
- Diagnose the nature and extent of any problem areas
- Offer constructive criticism when needed
- Identify areas for remediation
- Determine the effectiveness of the learning activities

Guidelines for providing effective feedback

Positive feedback affirms or reinforces the preceptee's clinical performance. For example, the preceptor observes as the preceptee admits a new patient and documents his or her assessment in accordance with established policies and procedures. The preceptor then tells the preceptee, "Congratulations! Your patient admission was done perfectly." Result for the preceptee:

- Affords feelings of success
- Enhances motivation for learning
- Reinforces desired performance

Negative feedback inhibits or modifies the preceptee's clinical performance. For example, the preceptor sees that the preceptee's admitting documentation is incomplete and states, "You did not document that admission correctly." Result for the preceptee:

- Tends to discourage and demoralize
- Limits or reduces motivation for learning
- Tends to focus on what not to do

It is important for preceptors to practice giving constructive feedback whenever preceptees need to correct or improve their performance.

Constructive feedback, like negative feedback, is intended to modify performance but, like positive feedback, conveys its message with supportive language. For example, the preceptor tells the preceptee, "I reviewed your admission documentation and found that almost all of the important areas were well documented. Because these areas were covered so well, I was surprised to find that no entries were made for the patient's allergies or medication history. Could you tell me why these were omitted?" Result for the preceptee:

- Enables him or her to experience at least partial success

- Maintains motivation for learning

- Reinforces desired performance and corrects unsatisfactory performance

B.E.E.R. feedback method

One technique for creating effective feedback is to use the following four-step model for criticizing and correcting behavior and performance problems. This model is based on a process that involves asking yourself questions about your preceptee's behavior. Remember the acronym "B.E.E.R.":

- **B:** Behavior—What is the employee doing or not doing that is unacceptable?

- **E:** Effect—Why is the behavior unacceptable? How does it hurt productivity, bother others, and so on?

- **E:** Expectation—What do you expect the employee to do or not do to change?

- **R:** Result—What will happen if the employee changes (positive tone) or this behavior continues (negative tone)?

Comparison examples of applied feedback

Once you have formulated your feedback, use the following rules as guidance on giving effective feedback to your preceptee.

Use descriptive rather than evaluative terms. Always make a conscious effort to describe both positive and negative behaviors. For example, the preceptor observes the preceptee greeting the patient correctly, giving her name, and stating that she will be her nurse for the day. However, she was not wearing her name tag.

- *Evaluative feedback:* "Your name tag is missing, and the manager won't like it!"

- *Descriptive feedback:* "You greeted that patient according to the unit guidelines. Can you think of anything that would help your patient remember you?" Have the preceptee use critical thinking to discover the problem.

Be specific rather than general in comments. For example, the preceptee learned how to successfully initiate IV therapy last week.

- *General anecdotal feedback:* "IV initiation skills acceptable."

- *Specific anecdotal feedback:* "Preceptee initiated three IV starts with a single attempt each time; aseptic technique used; patient stated that the process was comfortable."

Focus on your preceptee's behavior rather than on his or her personality. For example, the preceptee has been consistently late for the patient report at the beginning of the shift and disrupts the shift report when he does get there. The rest of the staff members have complained to the preceptor about the rude, disruptive behavior, saying the preceptee is inconsiderate.

- *Personality-based feedback:* "You have been very inconsiderate of the other staff members. They don't like you interrupting report."
- *Behavior-based feedback:* "You have been arriving at report late this week. Is there a problem arriving on time? When a staff member is late, it disrupts the flow of the report, and items may be missed. What can you do to ensure that you are here on time?"

Focus on sharing information rather than giving advice. For example, a patient's dressing change is due.

- *Giving advice:* "I think you (the preceptee) should do Mrs. Jones' dressing now. She is scheduled for therapy at 3 p.m."
- *Sharing information:* "I just got a call from therapy; Mrs. Jones is scheduled for 3 p.m. Is there anything she needs to have done before her appointment?"

Feedback should be well timed. For example, the preceptor observes a mistake in the preceptee's transcription of a physician's order.

- *Poorly timed feedback:* "You made a mistake and need to correct it," said while at the nurses' station and in front of the unit clerk.
- *Well-timed feedback:* Preceptor removes the chart to the break room and tells the preceptee privately, "You made a mistake and need to correct it."

Give your preceptee enough time to accept the feedback prior to making a plan that will involve change in behavior. For example, the preceptor observes that the preceptee consistently fails to listen to all areas of the chest when doing a respiratory assessment.

- *Impatient preceptor feedback:* "You consistently fail to listen to all areas of the posterior and anterior chest when doing your respiratory assessment. What are you going to do about it?"

- *Patient preceptor feedback:* "You consistently fail to listen to all areas of the posterior and anterior chest when doing your respiratory assessment. Please review the assessment process in your text and get back to me tomorrow about how you can use this information to improve your skills."

Avoid "ganging up" or giving the impression that you and other staff members are ganging up on your preceptee. An example is when staff members complain that the preceptee is taking too much time to complete his or her charting.

- *Ganging-up approach:* "The staff and I feel that you are spending too much time with patients and not enough time completing your charting."

- *Alternative approach:* "I have observed you spending a lot of time with patients, but your documentation has not been complete. How can you complete your charting and still spend needed time with your patients?"

Whichever approach you use in providing feedback to your preceptees, these guidelines are important to consider. Discuss them with your preceptee, the manager, staff, and educator as you define the parameters of the preceptorship. Will feedback be shared? For example, will the preceptee keep a journal and use it as part of the feedback process in reflective discussions with you when assessing his or her progress? How will the feedback be used to support and encourage the preceptee? How is it used to correct and counsel? How will the feedback be used to measure the preceptee's progress toward independent practice and transition to service?

Consistent, accurate, and respectful feedback is critical to the success of every preceptee and preceptor. Be sure to elicit feedback in your preceptor role, as well, to remain in alignment with your preceptoring agreement and the needs of your preceptee. Such feedback contributes to your own continued development and is important to build your own knowledge, skills, and abilities as a specialist in preceptoring.

Performance Evaluation Process

The better a man is, the more mistakes he will make,
for the more new things he will try. I would never promote
to a top-level job a man who was not making mistakes....
Otherwise he is sure to be mediocre.
—Peter Drucker

Performance evaluations facilitate preceptees' learning and success-ful transition into their new practice settings. They should be affirming and future oriented. As each required competency is successfully demonstrated, tell your preceptee an objective has been completed. Review the documentation form each day and check off the day's accomplishments.

You can best identify and communicate progress through feedback and evaluations—and mistakes. How can the mistakes you and your preceptee make be managed safely and successfully? Perform-ing regular evaluations can help you and your preceptee review mistakes through reflective discussion, for example, and identify appropriate or needed changes. Can mistakes measure your ability to delegate tasks? Can they assess the preceptee's ability to take on increasing responsibility? How can mistakes be used positively?

Let's look more closely at the nature of mistakes and see how they benefit you and your preceptee.

Mistakes can be a measure of ability to take on responsibility

Mistakes are an important part of the growth process for preceptors and preceptees. Maxwell (2000) describes how necessary it is for preceptors and preceptees to be able to recognize the importance of making mistakes, accepting responsibility for wrong actions, attitudes, or decisions, and learning how to keep mistakes in perspective. *MISTAKES* are

- Messages that give feedback about life
- Interruptions that cause us to reflect and think
- Signposts to direct us to the right path
- Tests to push us toward greater maturity
- Awakenings that keep us mentally engaged
- Keys we can use to unlock each door of opportunity
- Explorations to let us journey where we've never been before
- Statements about our development and progress

It is important to communicate to your preceptee those areas that need further experience or improvement. Be direct and address negatives first. Do not sandwich negatives between two positives; that approach dilutes the effectiveness of both. Not all criticism can be positive. Do not be apologetic about constructive criticism. As a preceptor, you have a responsibility to require good performance and the ability to facilitate it.

Collaborate with your preceptee to develop a plan to take safe risks and "fail forward," try new things, and improve these areas. Areas for improvement must be discussed as they are identified. Assess how the preceptee approaches negative experiences.

Maxwell (2000, p. 8) describes the different ways preceptees respond to mistakes by *failing backward* or by *failing forward,* as compared in the two lists below. Preceptors and preceptees must be able to handle mistakes by failing forward to successfully meet the challenges encountered in any new position or set of responsibilities. Keep your manager updated on any areas that do not progress as expected.

Failing backward	Failing forward
• Blaming others • Repeating the same mistakes • Expecting never to fail again • Expecting to continually fail • Accepting tradition blindly • Being limited by past mistakes • Thinking I am a failure • Quitting	• Taking responsibility • Learning from each mistake • Knowing failure is part of progress • Maintaining a positive attitude • Challenging outdated assumptions • Taking new risks • Believing a process or system didn't work • Persevering

End-of-orientation evaluation

There should be *no* surprises at the end of the orientation or at the close of the formal preceptorship program. Select an appropriate setting to review and discuss the final performance evaluation summary. Consider the following guidelines:

- Select a quiet, controlled environment without interruptions
- Maintain a relaxed but professional atmosphere
- Put the preceptee at ease
- Review specific examples of both positive and negative behaviors, activities, and attitudes
- Discuss future needs and goals

Express confidence in the preceptee's ability to do the work (unless there is good reason not to, which you should have already addressed in previous feedback sessions). *Do not* be hesitant in your encouragement of the preceptee's abilities, as appropriate. Be sure to:

- Be sincere and constructive in both praise and criticism
- Ask the preceptee how the preceptor (you) and clinical educator and/or nurse manager can improve the preceptorship

Initiate the peer relationship for preceptees and communicate this change in status to unit team members. Celebrate their transition into their new roles with a recognition ceremony, certificate of completion, or lunch, for example. Use any strategy to commemorate preceptees' change of status and welcome them to the team.

Mistakes are an important crucible for growth and forward movement. How do you find a way to engage one another positively in applying what is learned from mistakes to measuring progress toward transition to service? This can challenge any preceptor or preceptee. Changing how we look at mistakes and the potential they offer is the first step.

Confronting Reality Shock

If you are always worried about how you are performing a task, about how others perceive your performance, you will never perform it well. Performance requires forgetting yourself.
—Richard Saul Wurman

One of the major problems for healthcare institutions is the loss of new staff during the first six months of their employment. This group is made up of new graduates as well as seasoned professionals who are disillusioned with the modern healthcare environment. This disillusionment is commonly known as "reality shock" and can generate multiple mistakes and opportunities as preceptees find their way into the organization and new practice settings.

New nurses enter their assigned practice settings eager to begin their new jobs, to meet their new colleagues, and to accept their new challenges. They complete orientation and their competency verifications without difficulty. Their preceptors ease the transition into practice and teach them everything they need to be successful. Then, three months to a year later, disillusionment sets in. The preceptee realizes the new healthcare environment is flawed.

The phases of reality shock

There are four phases to reality shock. They are as follows:

1. **Honeymoon phase.** Preceptees are happy to be in their clinical rotations/finished with school/starting a new job. They perceive the new practice setting and their new coworkers positively, or through "rose-colored glasses." When asked, they may say, "Everything is wonderful!" During this phase, preceptees are actively focused on developing their own skills, mastering work routines, and meeting new people.

2. **Shock phase.** Preceptees begin to encounter weaknesses, discrepancies, and inconsistencies in the work environment and their new colleagues:

   - Coworkers with weaknesses—disorganized, tardy, or inattentive to duties

   - Lack of supplies, poor equipment maintenance, communication breakdown, or other obstacles to providing excellent, or "textbook," nursing care

   - Potential inconsistencies in expected professional nursing behaviors

   - Any situation that can cause frustration, anger, embarrassment, or disillusionment, such as being humiliated by another nurse or physician

3. **Recovery phase.** Preceptees begin to perceive the realities of the professional practice environment with a balanced view of both negative and positive aspects. They establish expectations that are consistent for all coworkers. The perspective that not all healthcare providers conform uniformly to the professional or organizational standards for conduct must

come from within the work setting. Once they achieve this, preceptees recognize their own fallibility. Their sense of humor may return during this phase.

4. **Resolution phase.** Caution! Preceptees may adopt less-than-ideal values or beliefs to resolve the conflicts of values and find ways to "fit in" with their new coworkers. Preceptors must help them retain the positive aspects of both values and belief systems—those taught at school and those held by practicing nurses.

How do you, as the preceptor, work within each of these phases to ensure that reality shock does not lead to resignation or adoption of poor values?

Ways to assist preceptees through workplace acclimation

There are many methods, strategies, and approaches for assisting preceptees through the various phases of reality shock. You work with your preceptees at their level of skill and performance to decide on the best ways to help ease them through each phase, such as those presented in the following examples.

Honeymoon:

- Develop the bonds between preceptors and preceptees, created by a mutual sense of trust, respect, and honor
- Harness their enthusiasm for learning new skills and routines
- Be realistic, but do not stifle their enthusiasm
- Introduce them to new staff and coworkers

Shock:

- Anticipate that preceptees may experience some dissatisfaction with new positions/peers/employers
- Listen attentively
- Model the ideals of professional nurses
- Help preceptees find appropriate supplies and functional equipment when needed
- Provide opportunities to vent frustrations in a constructive manner

Recovery:

- Always treat preceptees kindly
- Help them view situations realistically
- Ask them to keep a journal of improvements they would like to suggest and what outcomes they expect or would like to see
- Help them recognize positive aspects of their current work settings, as well as areas where improvements might be made
- Ease them into their roles and responsibilities; do not release preceptees to take full patient assignments until ready
- Protect them in times of adversity
- Always speak kindly about nurses and other healthcare providers
- Help preceptees regain their sense of humor

Resolution:

- Identify and manage any conflicts and confusions that persist
- Assist them in constructive and creative problem solving
- Describe mechanisms and processes available to resolve perceived problems or confusion

- Give simple, easy-to-follow directions for tasks
- Help them combine the best aspects of their prior school or work expectations with their current work situations
- *Caution:* Help preceptees retain the positive aspects of their nursing values/belief systems from school and from the practicing nurses

In summary, to help your preceptee move through the phases of reality shock, a balanced view of the workplace must be presented. It is especially important to recognize when your preceptee is moving toward the shock phase. Continue with open communication and consistent feedback. Here again, open honesty regarding the nursing unit, service, and organization must be held. The expression of genuine feelings and your own stories and real-life anecdotes about situations you have faced, actions contemplated, mistakes resolved, and outcomes achieved show your preceptees they, too, can learn from mistakes, overcome obstacles to professional practice, pass through the phases of reality shock, and successfully transition into service.

Letting Go

*If you are leaping a ravine, the moment of takeoff is
a bad time for considering alternative strategies.*
—John Cleese

"Letting go" begins with the welcome; in fact, part of the initial
planning for every preceptorship is the termination. Most organizations have time-limited orientations and clinical periods for
competency assessments and verifications for new hires. New
graduates may require additional time, which is negotiated during
the feedback sessions as the orientation unfolds.

Watch for some of the following indications that your preceptees
are ready to disengage (let go) from the preceptorship and take on
the increased responsibilities of being a staff nurse:

- Evidence that preceptees will not overlook important tasks
  related to the staff nurse role
- Demonstration that they can apply past clinical experiences to
  current ones
- Recognition of their own limitations of knowledge or skills
- Evidence of critical-thinking skills in the questions they ask

- Actively seeking more challenging experiences and greater autonomy in assignments

Keys for successful disengagement

Disengagement from a preceptorship opens the door to a mentoring relationship. Movement toward a peer role and potential mentorship requires the following three keys to be successful:

- Set expectations for all future performance, outlining the steps needed for all performance activities
- Motivate preceptees by focusing on strengths, releasing preceptees' potential within the organization
- Help preceptees find their "best fit" within the unit and organization

Consider celebrating the transition from preceptor to peer or mentor or both. Bringing tangible closure to the preceptorship can act as a rite of passage into the new staff nurse role with great expectations and equal measures of humor and resolution. Sometimes a preceptor and preceptee will form a particularly strong bond, one that will allow the preceptor to eventually become that preceptee's mentor. For example, this may occur when the once preceptor moves into a leadership or educator role and the previous preceptee wants to move into a similar role or position. Mentorships can grow from multiple contexts and reach across years.

For now, celebrate the completion of the preceptorship, leave the door open for new relationships and possibilities, and let go. As a preceptor, you have done your best. In letting go, you allow your now former preceptee to begin to do his or her best. It is now time to enjoy your new relationship as peers and coworkers.

Important Contacts

_____

Notes
_____